# The Author

Christina Weiser worked as an elementary school teacher for more than ten years before resigning her job and skipping off into freedom. She is an Ernst Fritz-Schubert-trained happiness teacher.

One day on her way to work in 2014, Christina broke five bones in her foot. For several months it was unclear if her foot would stay numb for the rest of her life. It was during this time that Christina decided to become healthy again. More than just recover, Christina decided that she was going to use her two healthy feet to realize her long-time dream of traveling around the world for one year.

With a lot of patience, positive visualization, the help of good doctors and caring people and her firm belief that she would soon be standing with two healthy feet in flip-flops at the other end of the world, Christina's foot healed in one and a half years.

For years she suffered from anxiety and panic attacks. But with a lot of work and a strong will, she learned to live with her fears. Some, like her fear of flying, disappeared completely.

During her time as a teacher, Christina worked with a child suffering from cancer. She often contemplated the condition of her student and felt like he should be learning something more meaningful than just Math or German.

So on occasion she would cautiously incorporate happiness activities into her curriculum to provide her student with additional psychological support. This experience played a role in the creation of this book.

There were times after her accident when, as Christina laid hopelessly in bed, imagining living the rest of her life with a numb foot, she too could have used a book like this.

Today Christina Weiser the person, author, world traveler and yoga instructor is at home traveling the world and loves to inspire people and give them a small gift of happiness.

With this book she would like to give courage to all those people suffering from a physical or psychological illness or injury. Her goal is to provide loving, empathetic and practical support that leads to self-love in both the good and most difficult of times.

# Get well!

*Actively design a happier life during your period of recovery*

Christina Weiser

# Dedication

## To mom and dad

Thank you for loving me since the moment I was born, caring for and appreciating me and teaching me how to love.

Without you, I would not be able to love.

You gave me the roots of love!

I love you!

## To Micha Hilgers

You helped me to rediscover my capacity for self-love and taught me to take responsibility for myself and my life.

Without you, I would not be the human being that I am today.
You lent me the wings that I needed to fly!

I thank you with all of my heart!

Dear reader,

With this booklet I would like to help you proactively manage time during your recovery period so that it is easier and a bit happier.

In the next few pages I will tell you what this all has to do with self-love.

All you need is your eyes and an open heart.

If you'd like to get creative, put together a recovery book. Get a few colored pencils, glue, photos, newspaper clippings or other material (no, you don't need to "know" how to paint!) AND perhaps most importantly, choose self-love. You can also "just" read this book.

When you see the following image, you have room to write or be creative:

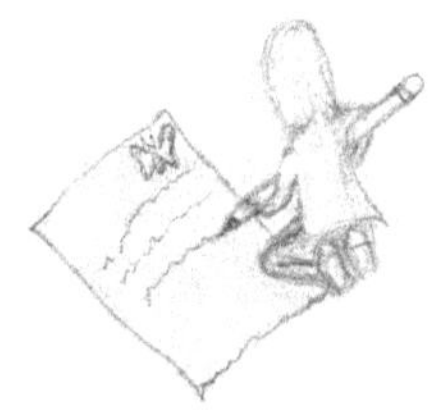

Only you can choose self-love.

Want to try?

Then give it a shot!

"Love is the strength,

that will help you escape the pain,

and nothing in life exceeds self-love.

If you feel deficient, helpless or lonely,

it always comes back to a lack of self-
love.

Take a moment to embrace yourself
spiritually and give

yourself the gift of love.

You deserve love, always."

(Unknown)

*Your Questions, Fears and Worries*

Are you injured or sick?

Feel exhausted?

Plagued by aches and pains?

Perhaps you don't feel well?

Or maybe you are facing surgery?

Are you afraid?

Are you full of worry? ...

I understand. In your situation it is completely normal.

I'll show you how you can get through your recovery period a little bit easier and sometimes even enjoy it.

The trick is called *self-love*.

Even if it might sound a bit strange to you at first, give it a try. You have nothing to lose!

I'm sure you have thousands of questions running through your mind.

Will I ever regain my health?

Will I be able to do all the things that I want to do again?

Will I overcome all of this?

Who will take care of me?

Who will take care of my family/ pet(s)?

How can I deal with everyday life?

Will I ever be completely healthy again?

Can they get by without me at the office?

How can I get these thoughts out of my mind?

Questions that you may have already asked yourself.

*The good news:*

Even if you feel powerless at the moment, there is something very important that you can do to get healthy:

*Give yourself the gift of self-love –*
*and as much as possible!*

What you need more than anything right now is self-love, trust, moments of happiness, positive thoughts and help from caring people.

Of course this doesn't mean that self-love alone can make you healthy again, but rather that it is an important ingredient in your recovery and an important foundation for living a happy life.

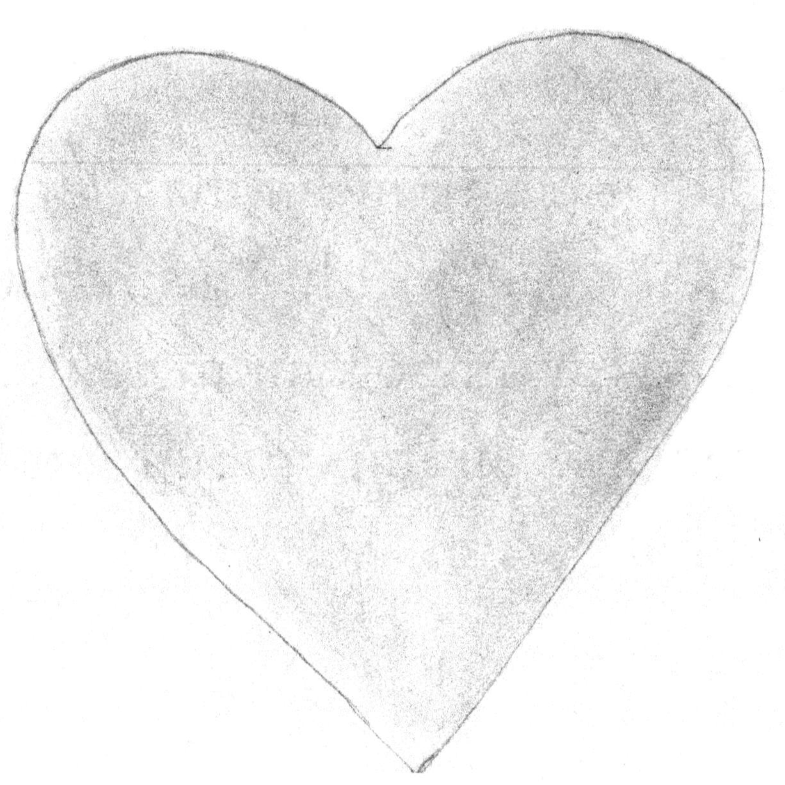

*Your Emotions*

Are you scared? Do you feel powerless or helpless?

These are completely normal feelings for somebody in your situation.

Without these kind of "negative" feelings like fear, anger, grief, or guilt, you would be a callous person.

Fortunately you are anything but that.

Some feelings (especially „negative" ones) we would often like to suppress or push aside.

Have you ever experienced this?

The problem is that these emotions do not "go away", but instead eventually grow stronger or end up impacting you in ways that you do not realize.

Fear, for example, only decreases when you accept it and let yourself feel it.


Sounds quite easy, I know, but I realize it isn't.

That said, I know that you can do it!

Be conscious. The fear is part of you, but the fear does not define you.


If you frantically try to push it away, it will only get worse and you don't want that either, right?

Instead, try to observe your emotions and really let yourself "feel" them without judging. If you accept your emotions, then over time they can become less irritating or bothersome. I know it's difficult, but it is definitely possible and these are skills that you can train especially well with meditation, yoga or breathing exercises.


Be conscious of your emotions.


Now all of your feelings are allowed to exist and they want to be seen.


You are so much more than just your emotions!

What do you feel? How do you feel?

Better yet, close your eyes and really try to understand what you are feeling inside.

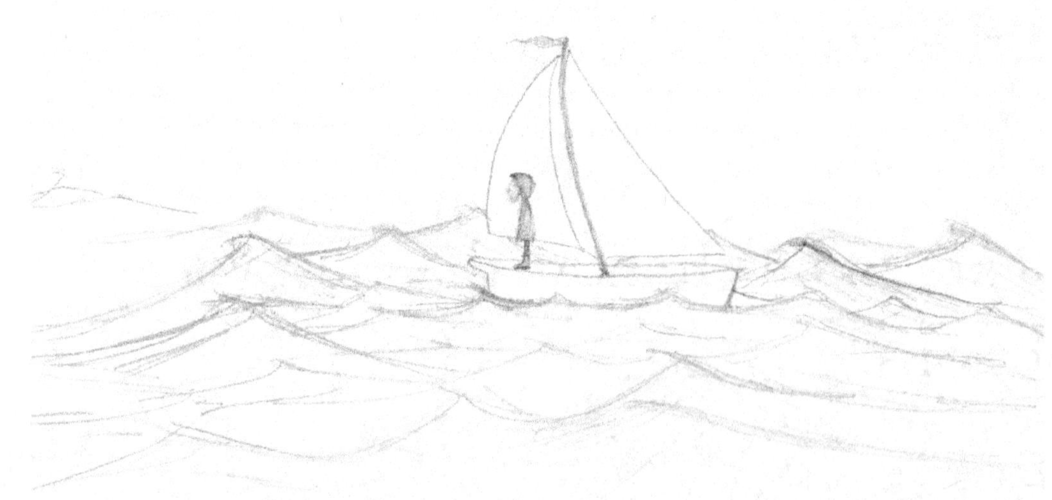

Angry?

Let it out!!!
(Without hurting anybody, of course.)

Punch your pillow 20 times (or more)!

Scream as loud as you can (not in anybody's ear, please)!
Let it out!

Scream into your pillow as loud as you can!

No better time than NOW!

…

Better?

Are you sad?

Cry.


Let the tears flow!

Let it out!


Your sadness also wants to be seen.
You don't have to suppress it.


After that you will certainly feel a bit
liberated.

# My Emotions

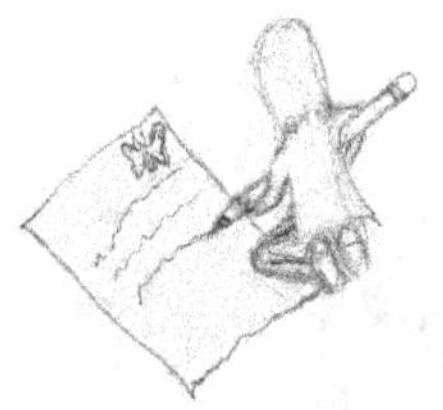

## Your Thoughts, Worries and Questions

Certainly you have thoughts, worries and questions that bother you.

Write them down. Get them off your chest!

The expression "get something off your chest" doesn't exist for nothing. Numerous scientific studies have shown that expressive writing can help heal the body and soul and even strengthen the immune system.

Give it a try!

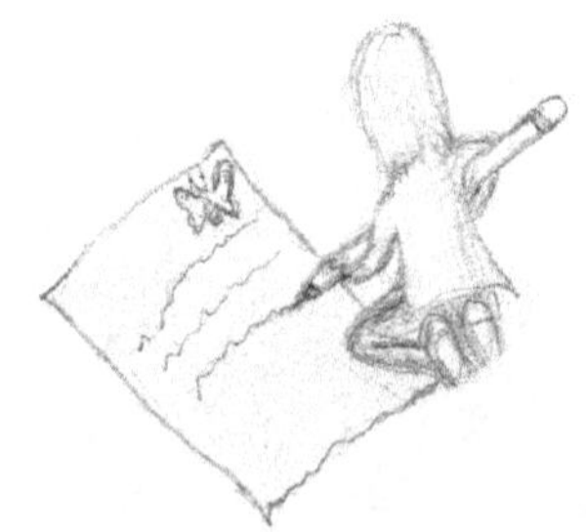

# My Thoughts, Worries and Questions

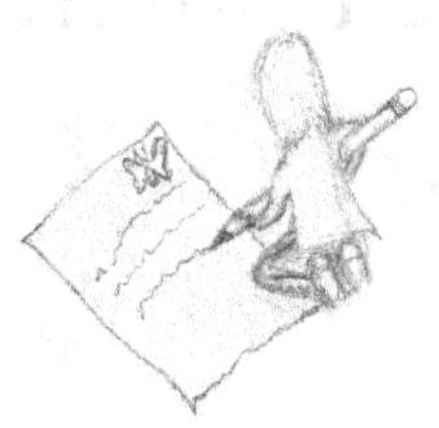

Share your questions, worries and fears with people that you trust, including your doctors, nurses and loved ones.

They are there to help you. Be courageous!

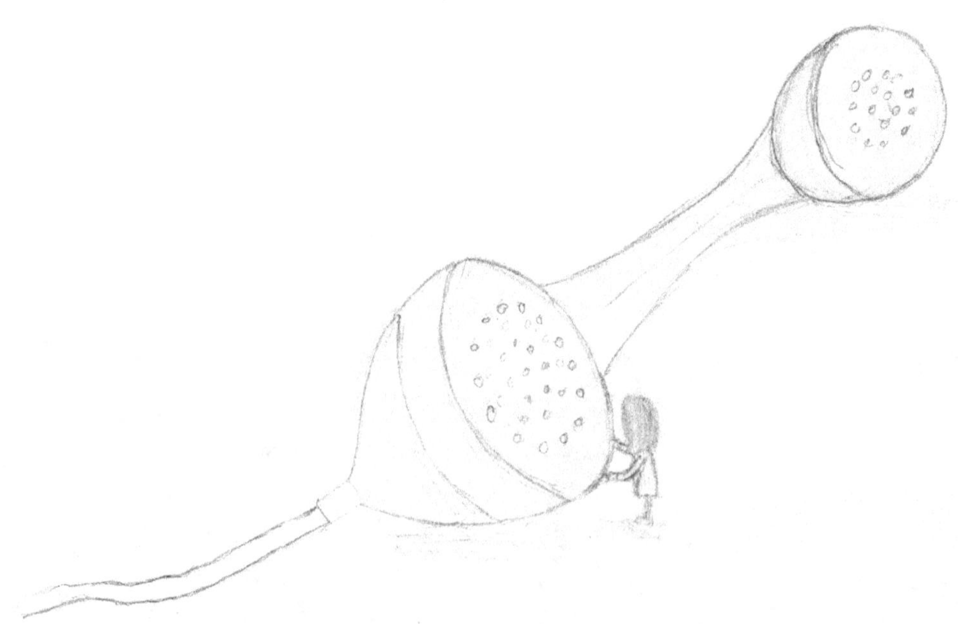

*Accept Help*

Practice accepting help!

Right now you need help at every turn.

Accept help and be clear about what you need!

This way you can fully concentrate on your recovery.

Let other people help you fulfill your needs and wants!

I need help with:

These ♥-people can help me:

*A Break for Body and Soul*

Now your body needs a rest.
Or maybe your soul needs a break.

As your body is inseparably linked to your soul, it automatically gets a break as well (or vice-versa).
Maybe it is even secretly celebrating.

Indulge in this break with all your heart.
YOU are the most important thing right now!
(By the way, it is not only in moments of illness or injury that you are the most important thing in your life, but ALWAYS!)

„From start to the end, we spend every second of our lives with ourselves. Isn't it worth it then to like and be kind to ourselves?"

(Unknown)

## ♥ *Self-Love Mantra*

Write down:

*„I am the most important thing in my life.*

*I deserve to treat myself well!"*

(Of course you are free to formulate this mantra
however you would like. The most important thing
is to find the words that make the biggest impact.)

_______________________________________________

_______________________________________________

_______________________________________________

_______________________________________________

Read this aloud every morning and evening
for the duration of your recovery (or even
better for at least 30 days beyond). Read it
as often as you can!

Maybe you are thinking:

"I am the most important thing in my life?

But there is also…

And I still have to …!"

NO! YOU are the most important person in your life. That doesn't make you egotistical. You are truly the most important person in your life. After that you can think about other people.

Maybe you have been taught otherwise, but the truth is only those who love themselves can stay healthy and help others.

But it's never too late to learn as your new outlook will also help you once your physical condition has returned to 100%!

Your body wants to be taken care of and so does your soul.

*Wertschätzende Selbstgespräche*

We often speak to others much more friendly and appreciatively than we do ourselves.

Can you relate?


This is often because we believe that there is something wrong with us the way that we are. But the truth is that you are exactly who you are supposed to be, just the way you are.


How do you talk to yourself?


Take note sometime.

Do you look down on yourself because of your illness or injury?

Are you prone to negative self-talk?

Now you have the chance to learn to speak to yourself appreciatively.
Do not blame yourself for your illness or slip into remorseful thinking.

Instead, consciously focus on your recovery and the fact that you are just fine the way you are and will soon be healthy again.

Perhaps the following self-love mantra will help.

 Self-Love Mantra

Write down:

*„I am just fine the way I am.*

*I deserve appreciative self-talk!"*

(Of course you are free to formulate this mantra however you would like. The most important thing is to find the words that make the biggest impact.)

_________________________________________

_________________________________________

_________________________________________

Read this aloud every morning and evening for the duration of your recovery (or even better for at least 30 days beyond). Read it as often as you can!

*Make Your Own Decision!*

Your body belongs to you and you only!

Thus you should be the only one who decides who cares for, operates on or supports your body. Same goes for your soul.

Find doctors and other people that you can fully trust and decide for yourself who you feel most comfortable with.

Be open to advice, but:

*You decide!*

*Trust*

It will certainly be of help to confide in other people.

Who do you immediately think of?
Who could help you the most right now?

🩶 Write down the names of the people below:

____________________________________________

____________________________________________

____________________________________________

____________________________________________

Ask these people to lend you an ear and then talk to them.

*Let Others Serve You!*

You can't avoid a hospital stay? Great!

"Great?", you might be thinking.

You probably find a hospital stay a truly horrible idea and I definitely understand that.

But take a step back and try to see it another way:

This is an opportunity to get help and let others serve you. You call the shots!

It's your turn to be king or queen for a change (you should try this much more often – while maintaining the dignity of those around you of course)!

This can sometimes be very therapeutic.

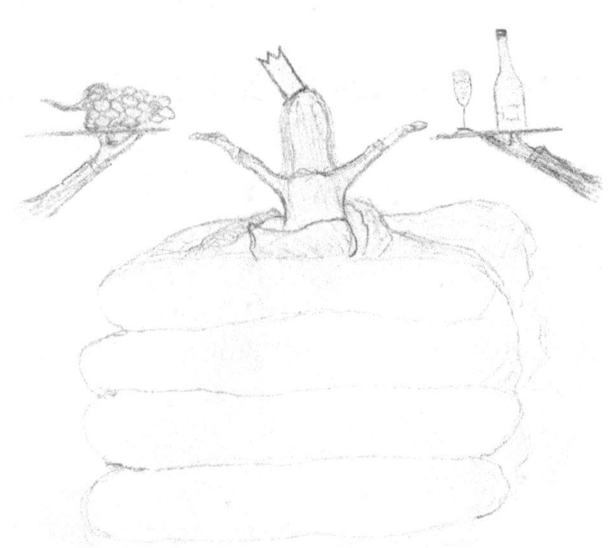

Perhaps you'll be in pain and in that case it is best to remain under the care of specialists who can properly treat you.

I understand that you would rather be at home, but is there somebody there to give you twenty-four hour care?

You'll be on your way home in no time.

Be sure that there are also loving people there to take care of you!

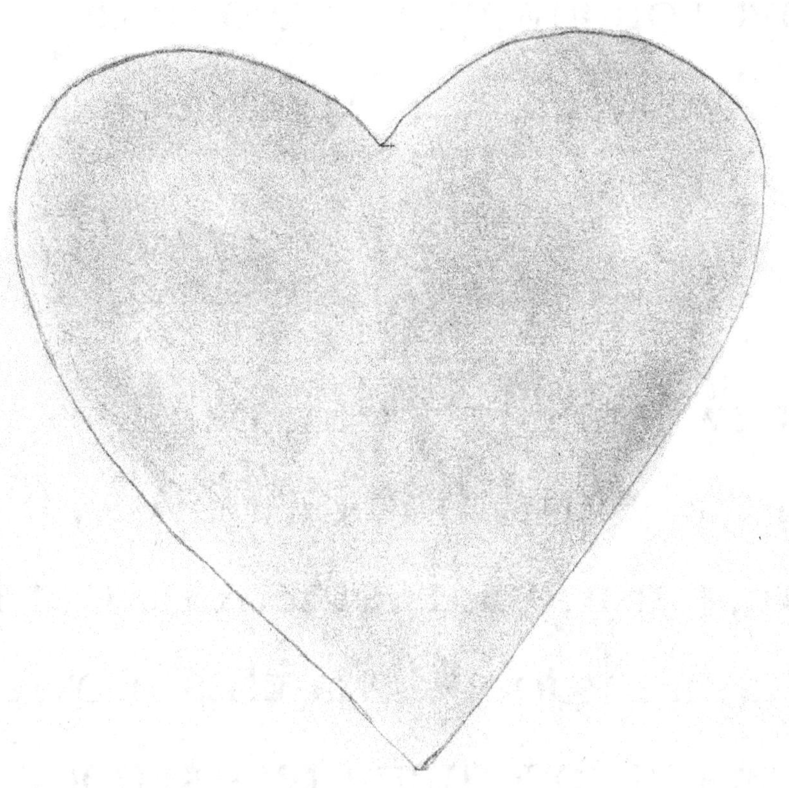

*Bored? Learn something new!*

Is the boredom really starting to get to you?

What have you always wanted to do that is now possible because of your current situation?

Learn a new language, knit, paint your nails, read an entire book (or two?), plan the future, paint, read something out loud, listen to an audiobook, watch a movie, do your taxes, put together a recipe book or maybe even write your own book?

Surely you can think of something?

Now you have the time to do it.

# Use it!

I always wanted to do/ learn this and
now I finally have the time:

_______________________________________

_______________________________________

_______________________________________

_______________________________________

# Do it! Get started!

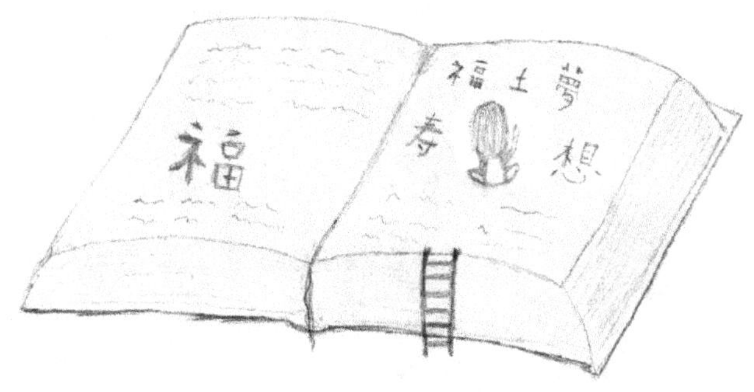

*Laughter is the Best Medicine*

Laughter releases anti-stress hormones and relaxes your muscles.

So what are you waiting for!

*Laughing Exercise*

Stand in front of a mirror (or hold one in front of your face/ ask somebody to hold one in front of your face) and smile for at least a minute.

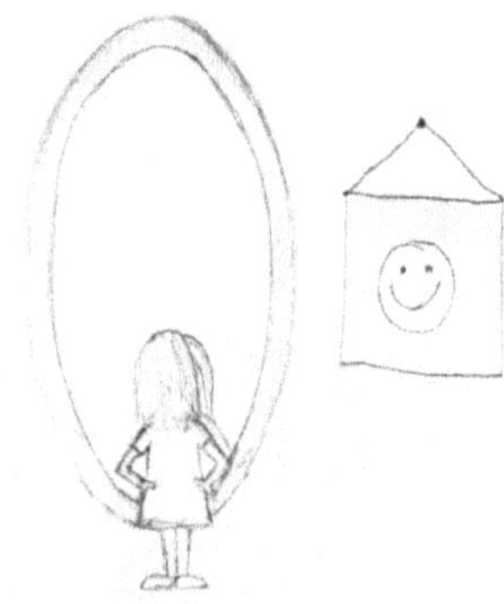

How do you feel now? ...

Better? Great!

Repeat this exercise every day as many times as you would like.

Invite people over who make you laugh, have somebody bring you a funny book or film or tell jokes with somebody!

*Fresh Kicks For You*

*Fresh Kick Tip No. 1*:  *Open the window!*

Take a deep breath and stretch out if you can!

Breathe in deeply through your nose and then out again through your mouth!

Repeat this three times.

If you can't stand up, ask somebody to open the window for you and follow the instructions above. This burst of freshness will serve you well!

Enjoy three times per day!

💗 *<u>Freh Kick Tip No. 2</u>: Rejuvinating skin wipes*

Ask somebody to bring you a facial wipe or moist towel and use it to freshen up!

It feels great!

## <u>*Fresh Kick Tip No. 3:*</u>  *Excursion*

Recharge with fresh air and nature!

If your condition allows, treat yourself to a trip through nature. Take a taxi or even better, go with somebody that you care about! It will give you a tremendous amount of new energy!

I hope that you are healthy enough to take advantage of this tip!

If not, take the trip in your mind and imagine how great it will be to experience it in the near future!

What do you say to a beach getaway?

Have somebody read the following beach getaway scenario out loud.

I wrote it for you.

## *Beach Getaway*

Make sure that you will not be interrupted for the next few minutes.

Position yourself comfortably in your bed and close your eyes if you would like.

Breathe in deeply through your nose and then out through your mouth. Then relax and continue breathing normally.

Imagine you are completely healthy.

You're strolling along a beautiful beach.

As you walk, the beach is slowly coming more and more into focus.

What do you see?

What do you feel?

What do you hear?

You feel the warm, soft sand beneath your feet.

It feels so good!

You let your gaze wander as you glance at the massive sea beside you. The warm sun is shining down on your face as you watch it reflect brightly off of the water's surface.

You stop, breathe in the fresh air and marvel at the beauty and depth of the sea.

Enjoy as much fresh air as you would like!

Each time you breathe out you feel more
and more relaxed.

You look into the liberating waves of the
sea.

Perhaps you lose your worries and fears in
the depths of the sea.

You listen to the waves as they rise and fall.

Your breathing is as steady as the rhythm of
the waves.

You walk further and discover a huge hammock that is stretched out between two palm trees.

You lay down and release your weight into the support of the hammock.


A light summer breeze lightly touches your skin.


Now you can completely let go.

You feel the warm sun rays tickle your skin as you enjoy the effortless support provided by the hammock.


You feel safe, relaxed and alive.

The peaceful sound of the waves relaxes you even further.

You are fully healthy as you lay in your hammock and enjoy the moment.

Each time you breathe in you get a rush of new energy. Each time you exhale you let go even further as you slip into a deep state of relaxation.

Enjoy it for a while.

Listen once more to the sound of the waves.

Feel the warm sunshine and the gentle sea breeze.

Breathe in the fresh air one more time.

Feel the rays of sun again as they warmly touch your skin.

Imagine them giving you new energy. This new energy slowly spreads throughout your entire body.

Take as much as you need!

Slowly you imagine sitting up in your hammock as you enjoy the sea view and sparkling shine of the water one more time.

You slowly climb out of the hammock as you take a step back and stand relaxed as you glance one more time around the beach.

Slowly bid farewell to your beach paradise and, at your own pace, come back to the here and now.

Move your hands and feet very slowly; shake them lightly to assist the circulation if you can. Move your fingers, stretch out or yawn; whatever helps you come back to the here and now.

Slowly open your eyes when you are ready.

Enjoy your new energy and state of relaxation.

Dream as often as you would like of being
back at your beach paradise!

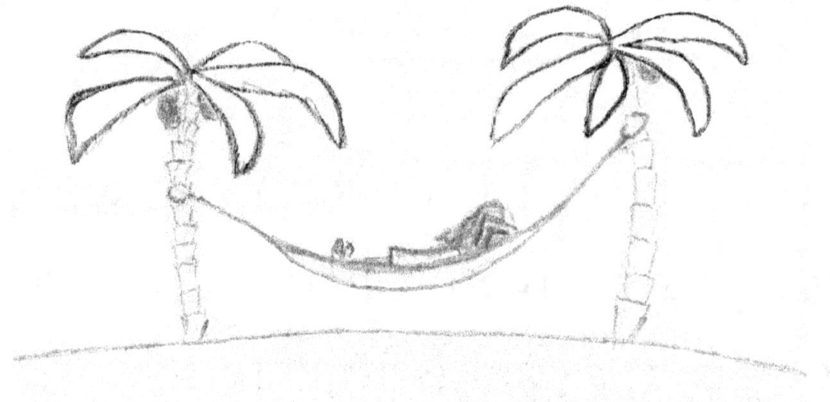

*Regain Strength*

Have you ever been to Bali?

Have you ever seen photos of their bright green rice fields?

To me these beautiful, light green fields stand for new strength, energy, growth and life.

Bali is my island of strength and healing, balance and self-love, life and growth.

I lived (in the truest sense of the word) there for nearly five months. The bright green of the rice fields injected so much new energy and strength into my life.

Perhaps you'd like take a mental trip to these magical, energy-infusing, green rice fields to regain some strength?

Then come and check out my website:

*www.christinaweiser.com*

*Be good to yourself!*

If a good friend or family member were sick or injured, you would also be patient and take good care of him right?

Then start taking care of yourself and treat yourself to something amazing!

Make sure you get sufficient sleep, healthy food and rest!

*I will treat myself to:*

*Your Favorite Dish*

Be sure to maintain a healthy diet; it is very important for your recovery.

If you don't have a special diet to follow, consider:

Who could cook something really delicious for me and what do I have an appetite for?

_______________ could cook

_______________ for me.

My Favorite Foods

# A Gift for You

Give yourself a gift!

What would you like?

A massage? A great book?

New music? A pleasant perfume?

Order it or have somebody bring it to you!

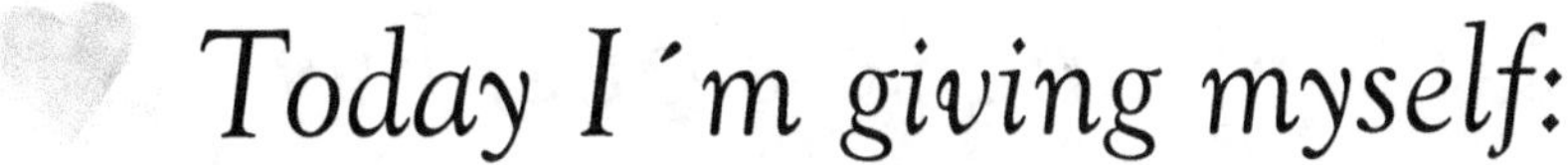 *Today I´m giving myself:*

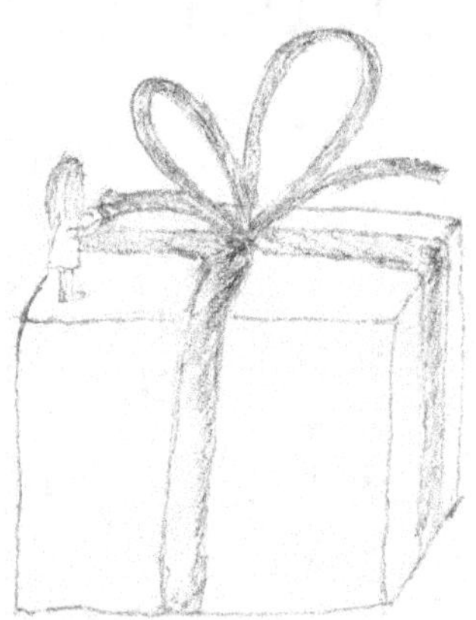

## Stay Fit

🩶    Stay fit (mentally and/ or physically) if you can!


🩶    For example you can do puzzles, read or learn a new language to keep your mind fit.

By reading this book or practicing self-love you are already on the right path.


If your condition allows, stay fit by performing short training sessions. Pay special attention that you don't overdue it, but don't let yourself get rusty either!


Please discuss your training program with your doctor before you begin.

## Set Healthy Limits

Perhaps you are receiving too many visitors and could really use more rest?

Then don't hesitate to let others know how you feel.

Communicate your needs very clearly and don't be afraid to sometimes say "No!"

A "no" often means a "yes" to you and can thus be very healthy.


Are you receiving too few visitors?


Kindly ask the people that you would most like to see to stop by.

*Think Positive!*

I know it is sometimes easier said than done and I'm not suggesting that you sugarcoat everything.

But try to get used to thinking positive and believing that you will soon be fit again.

Please don´t blame yourself if it doesn´t work out every day. Try to be kind to yourself!

Say (or even better scream) loudly:

*„I will get back in shape!"*

Close your eyes and picture it in your mind over and over again!

## Visualization: I Am Healthy

When I broke several bones in my foot a few years ago and the doctors told me that my foot could end up being numb for the rest of my life, I vowed to change my life. Every night I would lay in bed and think about the sabbatical year that I never had. I thought about my trip around the world that I had never gotten around to.

"My foot is probably going to be numb for the rest of my life? I'll never be able to wear high heels again? Not even to my wedding?", I asked the doctor in a horrified state as I sought a second opinion.

He looked at me and frowned.

"Well, maybe for a few hours...", he thought aloud.

I disagreed.

He prescribed an orthopedic shoe. Have you ever seen one of those things?

I inquired at a local specialty shoe store, imagined this massive block on my foot and decided: NEVER EVER!

I tore up the prescription and decided that I would get healthy and apply for my sabbatical year as I was determined to finally take that damned trip around the world as I had always intended, but never done.

My goal is not to encourage you to forego similar assistance devices or equipment. Please don't do that.

Instead, I would like to recommend a great technique: visualizing your desired condition.

I still remember when my good friend Jörg said to me, "Christina, imagine yourself fully healthy, doing one of your favorite activities!" (or something along those lines). To this day I am profoundly thankful to him as otherwise I would never have heard of this technique.

So I went back and forth between two images in my mind.

First, I imagined myself in high heels at my wedding. Then I imagined myself on my trip around the world, strolling through the sand in flip-flops with the sea by my side.

The visualization of my desired state helped me tremendously during my recovery and since then I have been fully convinced of the effectiveness of this technique.

The idea is to imagine yourself in your desired condition, fully recovered. To do this, you create images of your desired condition in your mind and, as emotionally as possible, you flip through them several times a day.

I have found this technique to be most effective when practiced in the morning, just after waking up and in the evening, just before going to sleep.

Between the occasional weeping session, I also listened at least three times per day to therapeutic meditations until I practically knew them by heart. I also went regularly to lymphatic drainage and acupuncture and visualized, over and over again, myself on the other side of the world in flip-flops.

Would you like to try it?


Then let's get started!

Have somebody read the text aloud or go to:

www.christinaweiser.com

There you can listen to the meditation for free.

*Visualization: I Am Healthy!*

Get as comfortable as possible and close your eyes.

Breathe in deeply through your nose and then out heavily through your mouth.

Afterwards, continue breathing normally.

Imagine you are completely healthy.

How do you look?

What are you wearing?

How do you feel?

Where are you?

Who is around you?

Are you talking to anybody?

What are you doing?

How do you move?

What is your demeanor?

Are you laughing?

What sounds do you hear?

Do you smell anything?

Do you see anything in particular?

Do you feel anything specific?


Enjoy the feeling of being completely
healthy and stay focused on this image in
your mind.


Let the image sink in; notice all the
wonderful colors!

And then breathe in deeply through your nose again and as you breathe out, let the image in your mind fade away.

Deepen your breathing as you let it drift past like clouds in the sky.


When you're ready, slowly move your wrists, fingers and feet and slowly bring your attention back to your physical location.


When you're ready, open your eyes.

Imagine your desired condition as often as possible and then let it go!

If you like, you can paint or write what you have seen. Paint or describe yourself with words; how you look when you are completely healthy again, or perhaps one of your favorite activities that you can't wait to do again.

# I am Healthy

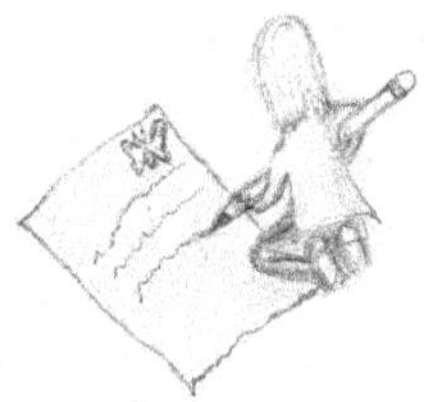

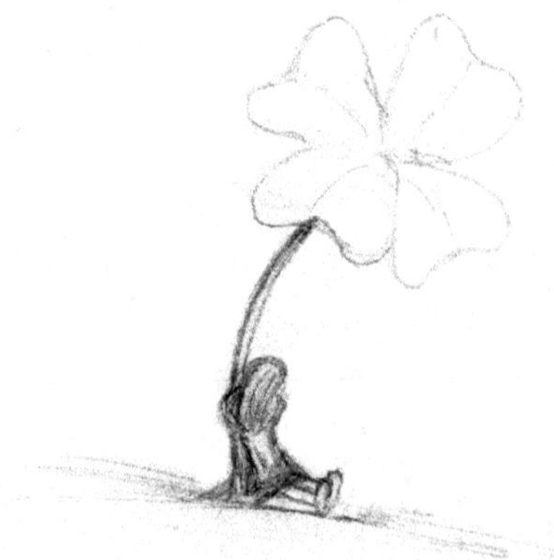

Here you can also paste a photo or collage of you performing this activity or even hang it near your bed!

"Transform
fear into drive,
worry into confidence,
resistance into acceptance,
anger into calm,
and problems into solutions."

(Unknown)

# Dream of Your Favorite Place

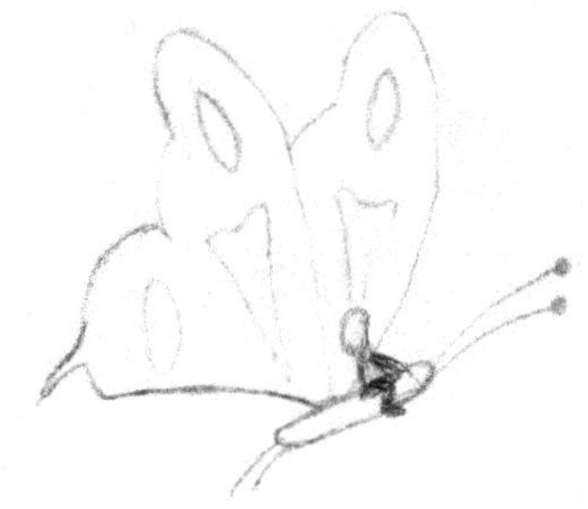

*Happiness Exercise*

Close your eyes and imagine your favorite place.

Where would you like to be right now?

What are you doing there?

Enjoy the time at your favorite place and let it fill you with new energy!

# My 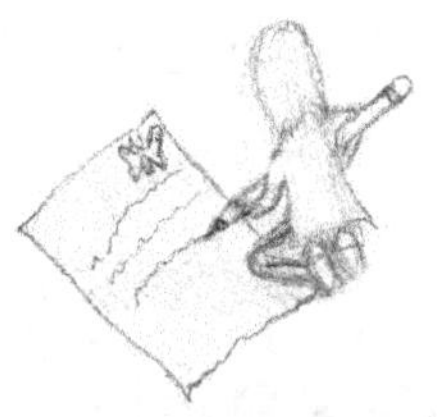 -place

# Feel-Good Music

Music is good for your ears and your soul.

What music would you like to hear?

What is your favorite song?

Do you prefer louder music or to relax with more peaceful tunes?

Turn it up? Dance? Sing along? Do it!

Turn the music up! It will liberate you!

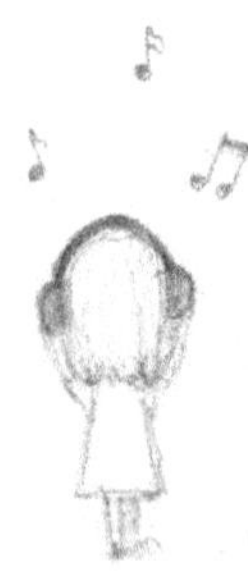

If you can't get up, you can sing loudly in bed. By the way, you can also dance while lying in bed (move individual body parts or simply use your imagination!) and even with crutches!

If you need to, my own experience has taught me that with a little practice, you can learn a few cool tricks (but please don't break anything…)!

Move your body parts to the rhythm of the music or close your eyes and relax if you need to rest.

Who could provide you some music?


My favorite music/ song:


________________


I will ask the following person/ people if he/ they can provide me with music:


________________


♡     Turn it up loud or enjoy the quiet melody!

# *It's O.K. to Hang Out!*

"Laziness is beautiful," my childhood hero Pippi Longstocking used to sing.

Even if you didn't really choose your laziness, it can still be "beautiful" or relaxing to just be lazy for a change!

Today I give you my official approval to just be lazy: You can be lazy!

Write as large as you want:

*I can be lazy!*

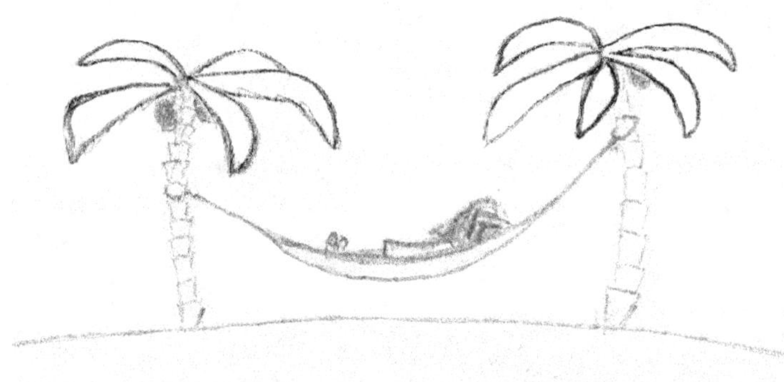

*Sense Yourself Within*

How am I doing? What do I need right now?

Stop a few times per day to just get a sense of how you are feeling within. Ask yourself, "How do I feel?"

Then you will immediately know what you need at any given time. This is an important element of self-love.

I feel...

I need...

I am doing...

I am looking for...

## *Relaxation*

Relax!

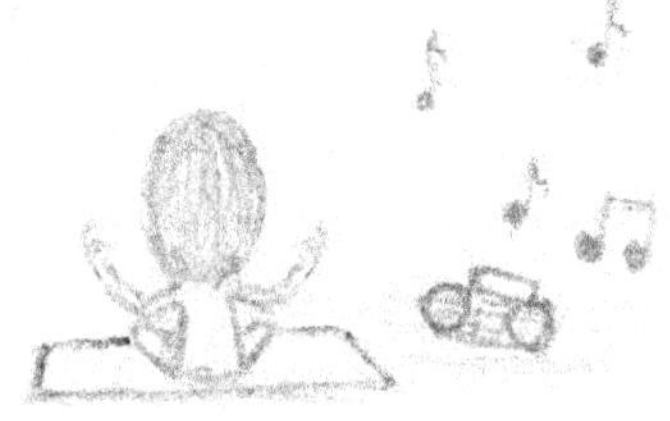 Consciously relax. For example, use a therapeutic meditation or imagine your dream vacation or whatever makes you feel good. It will build inner as well as physical strength.

Enjoy a cup of tea!

That pleasant warm feeling as the tea goes down your throat is simply amazing!

Or perhaps you'd prefer a cold beverage.

Then enjoy the refreshing feeling!

## Little Moments of Happiness

Even with the sorrow and difficulty of your current situation, you are certain to encounter a few moments of happiness each day, even if you don't immediately recognize them.

Perhaps somebody smiled at you today?

Did somebody help you?

Or maybe you took a small physical or mental step forward?

Are there people who are there for you?

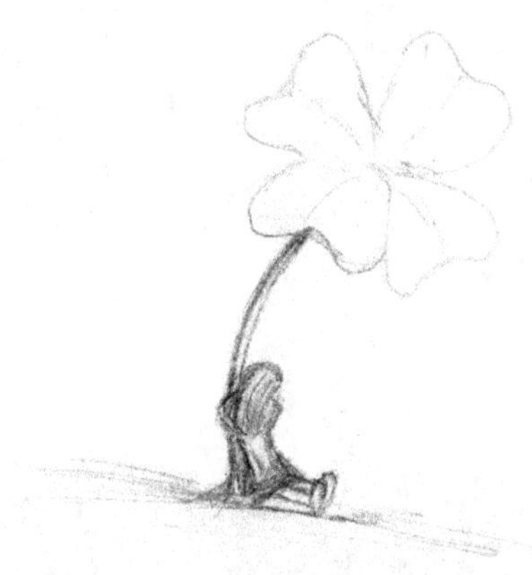

# My Little Moments of Happiness

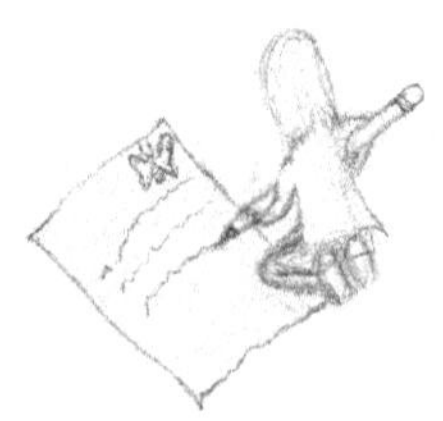

# My Goals

Your goals give you strength!

See them clearly! You will achieve them!

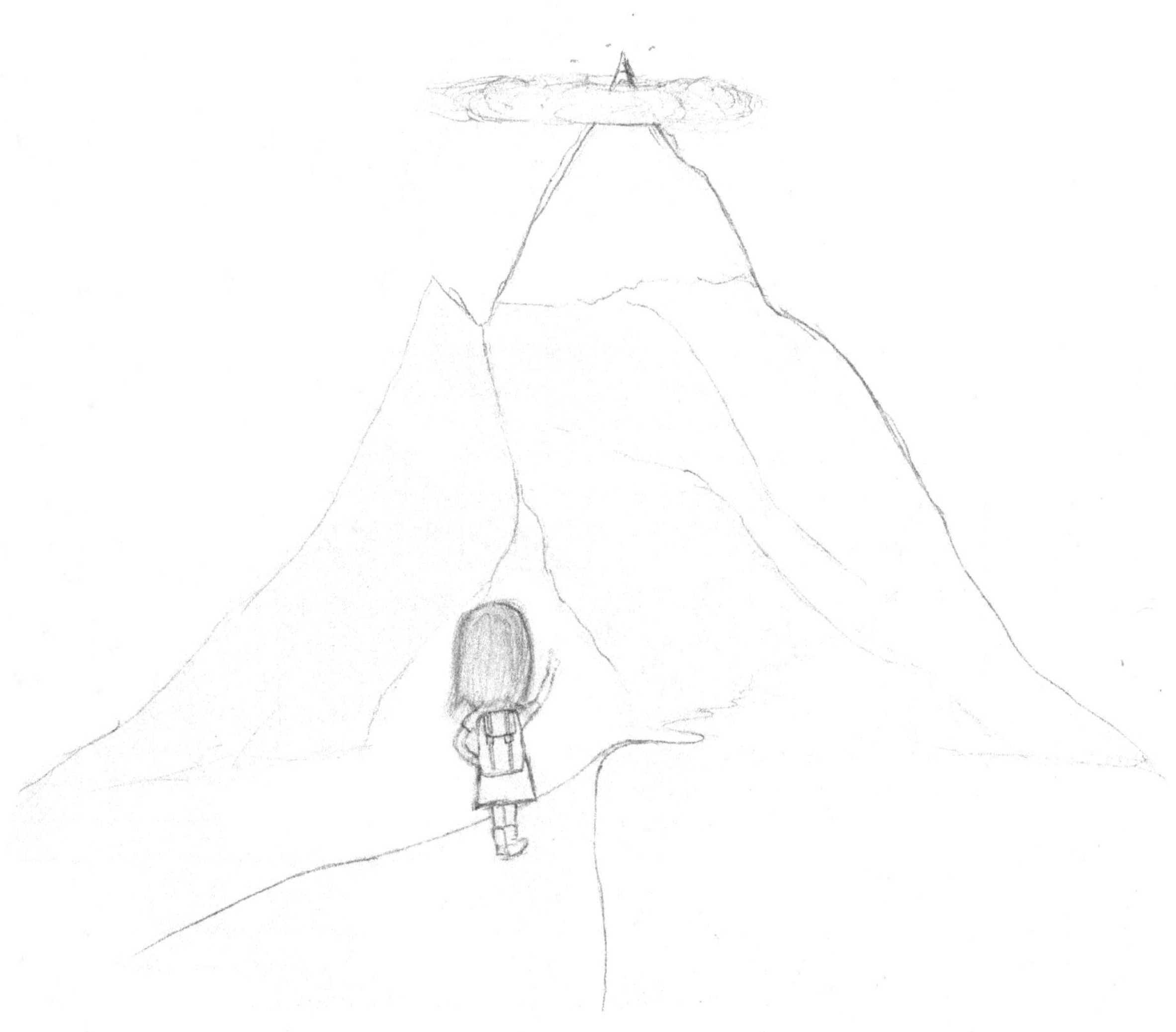

*I will soon be able to (once again) do the following*

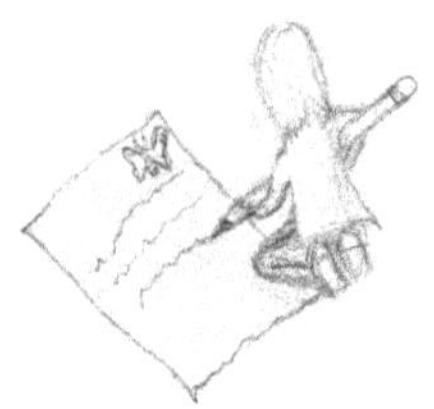

*Your Biggest Dream*


During my recovery period my dream trip around the world was constantly motivating me to regain my health.


Do you have a dream that has been dormant for a while?


Here you will find a place for it.


Make it known!


And then let it go!

# My Biggest Dream

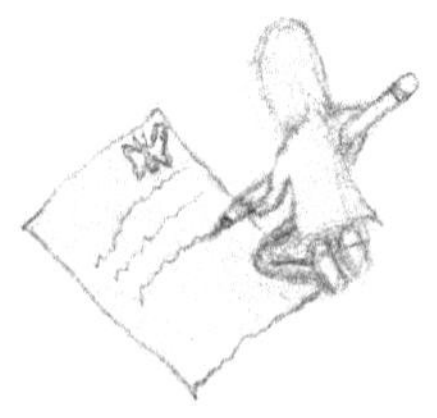

*Patience and Time*

Give yourself time to recover!

I know how difficult it is, but it is very important.

*"Have patience with all things and most importantly with yourself."*

(François de Sales)

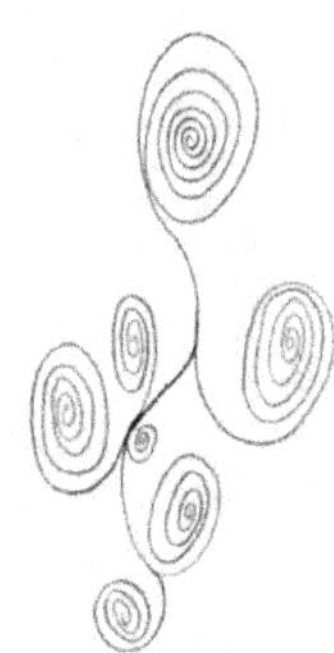

*Gratitude and Happiness*

Even in your current situation, gratitude can help you lead a happier life by making you conscious of all the things that you have to be thankful for instead of constantly thinking about what could be better.

What are you thankful for?

Each morning and evening jot down (or consider) at least three things that you are thankful for or little things that made you happy.

♥ You can even put together a small happiness booklet.


It can be very helpful to thank the people that you are thankful for!

# I Am Thankful...

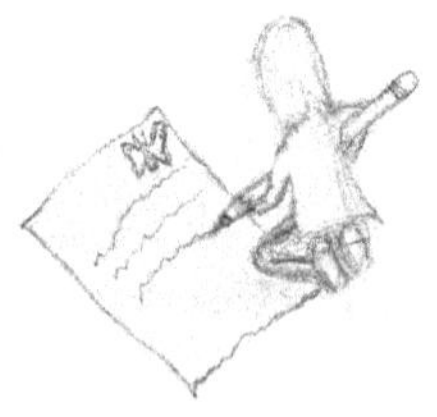

# I Am Happy...

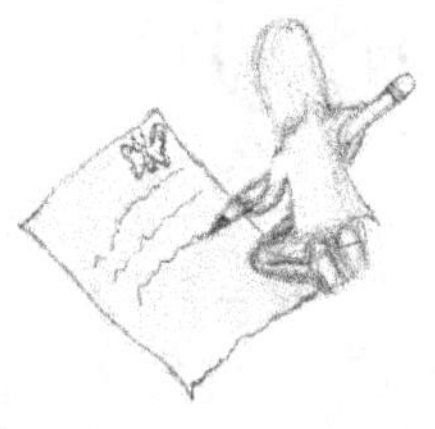

On your road to recovery I encourage you to never lose your courage. Give yourself the love that you deserve.

Give your body and soul the time they need to recover and be good to yourself!

I hope that I could give you a small bit of happiness and help you to actively incorporate happiness into your recovery period.


With love,

Christina Weiser

## *Thanks*

It has long been a dream of mine to write this booklet. And after letting it lie dormant on my laptop for far too long, I am excited to finally make it a reality.

I would like to thank everybody who has believed in me and given me strength.

You, along with some less than ideal experiences during my recovery, gave me the inspiration for this book.
When you are sick or on the other side of the world, you discover who is really there for you.

I thank my family that is always there for me with unconditional love when I need them. You have made me the person I am today; full of empathy and therefore capable of writing a book like this.

Thanks to my best friend Nadja, who always believes in and strengthens me, regardless of how crazy my ideas are.

I'd like to thank Micha Hilgers, who was the most amazing mentor that I could have hoped for on my road to health, self-love and freedom.

Thank you Dr. Graf Stenbock-Fermor, who as my trusted orthopedist, gave me endless courage and always supported me mentally, and with both conventional and alternative treatment methods throughout my recovery.

I'd like to thank Jörg Melchior who introduced me to the valuable idea of visualization. It changed my life.

I thank Claudius for the wonderful illustrations that have given a proverbial face to my words.

Thank you Jana and Manuel for formatting my book. After countless, nerve-racking hours of trying to do it myself and the failed attempts of an IT professional, they saved the book when I would otherwise have probably tossed it in the trash.

I want to thank Daniela for her patience and putting together such a lovely cover.

Thank you Jason for the wonderful translation into English.

I'd like to thank Dennis who always gave
me the inner strength to do what needed to
be done and to tell my story.

Finally, I would like to thank my readers for
sharing, gifting and promoting my book
and enabling us to help as many people as
possible.

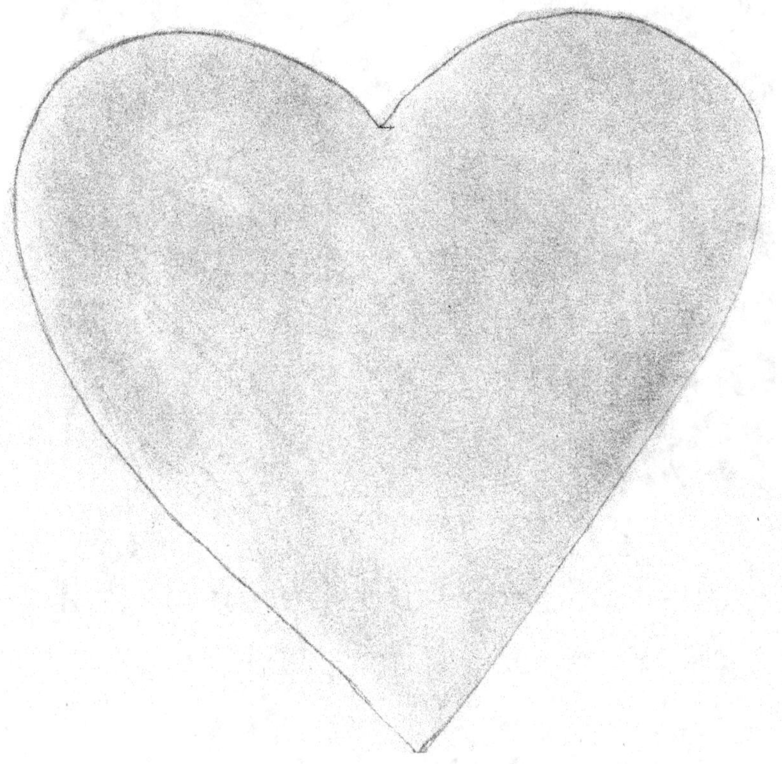

# Visit Christina Weiser on Social Media:

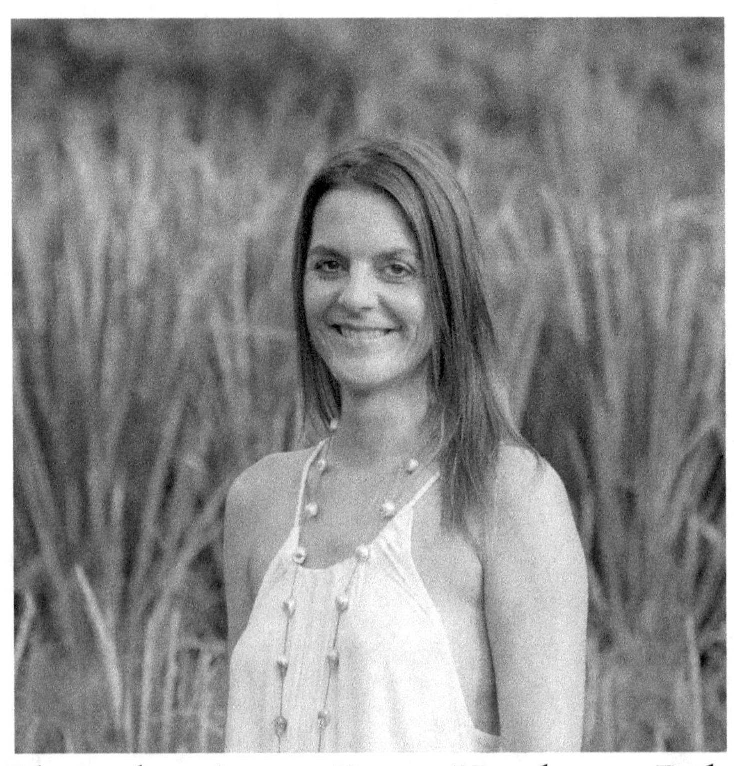

Photo by: Ageng Putra Kusdinar, Bali

www.christinaweiser.com
www.meervomleben.com
Instagram: christina.weiser
Facebook: Christina Weiser